MW01223545

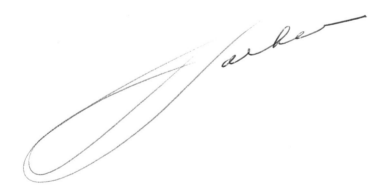

Louise,
MAKING LIFE,
LESS WORK
Jean

So.... So.... Clean!
IN JUST TWO HOURS A WEEK

(My Friend Kathy)

Photo by Cindy Lozza
Website: http://www.sosoclean.com

Printed in Victoria, Canada

A cataloguing record for this book that includes the U.S. Library of Congress Clasification number, the Library of Confress Call number and the dewey Decimal caltaloguing code is available from the National Library of Canada. The complete cataloguing record can be obtained from the National Library's online database at www.nlc-bnc.ca/amicus/index-e-html
ISBN: 1-4120-1293-7

LORHAN

This book has been Self-Published by the author in cooperation with Island Blueprint, 911 Fort Street, Victoria B.C. 250-385-9786

Dedicated to my life's crowning achievement, my three children; Paul, Alison & Shaun. And to my recently found birth daughter Tina and her family.

A special thanks to Judy Morten for the many hours she dedicated to editing.

CONTENTS

Chapter
ONE

KATHY HATES CLEANING

Chapter
ONE

The other day, a female acquaintance of mine was explaining the open wound on her hand, not a pretty sight, created by dry skin as a result of cleaning her bathrooms. Her story began; "I went home last night and thought I could clean my two bathrooms in 45 to 50 minutes if I worked fast and didn't get interrupted.........."

The story continued, but my mind went inward. I was in shock! If it takes her almost an hour to clean her bathrooms, how long does it take her to clean her whole house? I shook my head and returned to listening to the tale. I caught up with it somewhere near the end. This lapse could have been embarrassing if she had realized I had been paying very little attention after the shock of her opening statement.

If you find her estimate realistic, you are definitely wise in buying this book. What takes her and you so long? Do you get out the cotton swabs and clean between the tiles on the walls? You and I both know that when you pay enormous sums for an executive detailing of your car, they do exactly that: get out the cotton swabs and clean every little nook and cranny with exacting patience, extracting even the tiniest grain of dirt. And why not! You are paying for that exact intense kind of a job. But, think about this! Bathrooms are the two smallest rooms in your home and nobody is paying you even a paltry sum to clean them. I have two bathrooms with a combined total of 95 square feet. *I know this is an English measurement and it is a dead give away as to my age, but what can I say, I just don't relate to metric.* I have been in a lot of main bathrooms and many ensuite bathrooms, (*watch where your mind is going,*) over the years and I would say that my bathrooms are an average size. Considering that my place is 1154 square feet, if it took me an hour to clean my bathrooms, it would take me another 11 hours to finish cleaning the house. *Not on your life! As they say, life is too short.* Even before I developed my cleaning system, I never spent that amount of time cleaning.

The story, of course, is not important to the text of the book. The story was important to me as it germinated the idea to write this book. But, only partially! The other incentive had to do with my friend Kathy.

I have spent several hours on the phone, on more that one occasion, talking to my friend Kathy. Kathy was out of work and didn't have a job, a situation I had found myself in not more than a year previously. Without a job! A scary situation when you have to provide for your own livelihood. I was reminding Kathy that I had resorted to cleaning apartments in my condominium building when I was out of work. She thought this option was too embarrassing and degrading. Granted, cleaning homes for a living is not a psychologically comforting thought when you're used to executive positions! Our pride gets in the way, but it's my opinion, pride becomes a luxury you can't afford, when it comes to having a roof over your head and food on the table.

In any case, I did convince my friend Kathy to start this new adventure. I spent hours on the phone trying to explain my cleaning system. Now, my friend Kathy is not a genius nor is she lacking in intelligence; yet there were a lot of silences on the other end of the line. Do you suppose she hadn't a clue about what I was explaining? That was the case! I soon realized it was impossible to understand a verbal explanation of my Rotating Cleaning System, which I will refer to as **RCS** throughout the remainder of the book. It was apparent that I would have to document my system in black and white. Hence, Kathy is the second reason that convinced me to write this book.

I'm not yet finished with my friend Kathy's involvement with the book. She is also responsible for the third and deciding factor that brings this book to a reality.

Some people absolutely hate cleaning and I mean HATE. My friend Kathy is one of those people. Kathy Hates Cleaning! That sounds like a bumper sticker......**Kathy Hates Cleaning.** We could make up a bunch of bumper stickers....**Carolyn Hates Cleaning.....Judy Hates Cleaning.....Alison Hates Cleaning.** Let's face it, most people are not in love with the job of cleaning their homes, but it is a necessity. So, Kathy is like most of you she may hate cleaning, but she likes a clean home and this constant contradiction is a cause for a lot of mental anguish.

Kathy recently told me this story;
"I've made a deal," she said, "with a girlfriend, that if I die, she is to run over to my place and clean my oven and I will do the same thing for her." She added, "I don't want anybody to see my dirty oven."

If my oven was that dirty and it bothered me so much that I had to make such a morbid deal with a friend, I think I would just clean my oven and keep it clean. I don't think I would ever let it get to the point where it was so dirty I just couldn't talk myself into the task. If this sounds self-righteous, I apologize, but that is the way I think.

My **RCS** would allow Kathy to keep her oven clean without the trauma she associates with the job.

I have been trying for some time to get her to use my system, but to no avail. After hearing this death deal story, I am even more convinced that she should be using this cleaning system. It is to help make life a little easier for people like my friend Kathy that I write this book.

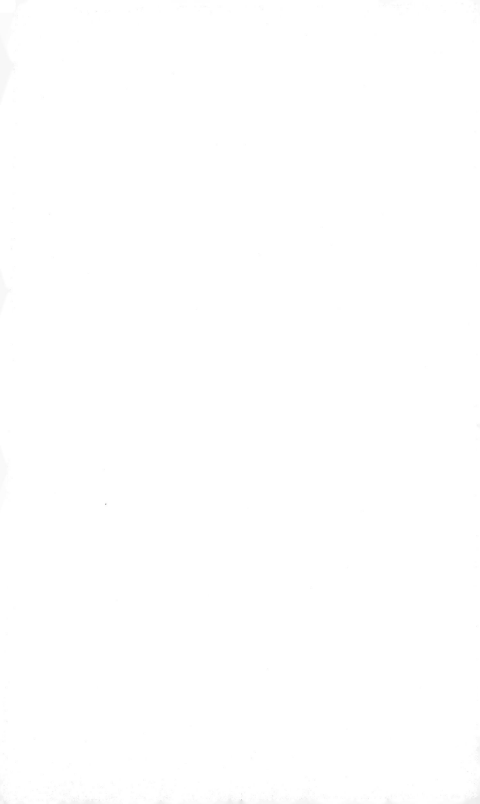

Chapter

TWO

THE WEEKEND

Chapter
TWO

I live in a two-bedroom condominium apartment, which I share with my adult son. I do the cleaning on Friday nights, so I can spend time doing the things I like on the weekends.

I still have vivid memories of years gone by, when every day was a workday. During those years I was working full time in a high powered, extremely demanding engineering position while bringing up three children and I shouldn't forget, a husband who, rightfully so, required some of my attention. In those days, I cleaned all day Saturday from the time I awoke until I went to bed. I was a perfectionist, a condition which age has thankfully tempered. On Sunday I would do six loads of laundry and the same evening do the ironing. I wonder today how I ever managed. *I know some of you can easily relate to this kind of schedule.*

If only I knew then, what I know today. I could have completed all my household chores in one day. Actually, my business at the time was managing major engineering projects. Don't let me mislead you; I didn't manage these projects alone, but my involvement certainly taught me how to schedule a multitude of items in order to reach a target date. In order to develop my **RCS,** I adopted the same principles that I used in business.

Consider the cleaning job as a project. Every project has a start date and a completion date. To effectively meet the end date, you must prepare a schedule of items to be completed within specific time frames. My **RCS** is designed to reach completion within two hours. The hardest part is getting started. If you have a schedule and know that you will complete the schedule within two hours, it is easier to get started. Even on my worst days I'm able to pull out my list, look at what I have to do and say, *"Okay! Lets just do it!"* Two hours later I have done the job. I'm a little tired, but feel good and I don't have to think about cleaning for another week. Anyone can cope with two hours of cleaning a week.

This past year, not one I wish to repeat, did yield at least one positive thing, an effective **Rotating Cleaning System**. This actually evolved after I acquired several units to clean in my building. I think I was becoming feeble minded because I couldn't remember from one week to the next what items I had to clean in the different units. In the course of preparing the schedule, it became blantantly obvious to me that I was over cleaning, as in too often, some items and not cleaning other items as often as necessary. Some items will actually stay looking clean if you clean them once every eight weeks. (*Once you get the dust under control that is!*) Preparing the schedule allowed me to ensure that all items were cleaned on a regular basis and without duplication. This organization saved me considerable time. As an example, one of my units took me 3 1/2 hours to clean when I first started and this same unit now takes me only 2 hours, and yes it is just as clean, probably more so, because nothing is overlooked. Everything is cleaned and cleaned again before most people would consider it dirty enough to clean. To clean something before it gets dirty sounds a little paranoid, but you will understand why as the book progresses.

Would you like a Friday, which is truly a T.G.I.F. day? As I said before, I'm a strong believer in the 'weekend'. We all deserve our downtime. This belief probably stems from my earlier days when there was no such thing as downtime. Most people I know today use their weekend to clean house, go to the grocery store, do the washing and ironing, mow the lawn, mend clothes, make repairs and so on. I get tired just thinking about such weekends and I can't figure out why people look forward to them, except for my son whose weekends are comprised of volleyball, squash, tennis, golf and partying. He has a cleaning lady-me! The plain truth is that most people finish their five-day job only to go to their two-day job, and then back to their five-day job. *Are you nuts? Isn't a five-day workweek enough?* Okay, so I know you're not nuts, probably just going nuts from this schedule. As you know, I used to do the same thing. I just didn't know any better.

Let's break the cycle. You already have to work five days a week. When I say this, I'm including those who go out to the workplace as well as those who stay at home. Believe me, I know how hard you work and for you I really do hope that you can break the cycle of working seven days. As long as you are in a work mode, by all means work, but only work the five days. Some with a very demanding schedule will work six. But for God's sake don't work seven. Even *He* took the seventh day to rest.

Give this idea some thought: washing - one-night; ironing - one night; groceries on the third night; cleaning "remember it will only take you 2 hours" on the fourth night and those extra chores - the fifth night. Sound impossible? Most of you spend your evenings now puttering. This energy just needs to be harnessed. Think about it! Most chores only take 2 hours or less and none of them are back breaking. Just 2 hours each night then you can foresee a glorious weekend to do as you wish! Now, for some, I know weekends are not totally free days, but let's hope the organized workload helps make them more enjoyable with some free time for you. This book is going to save you hours;

try to utilize them to your advantage. You have the choice.

You owe yourself at least one day off from work a week. Think of all those things that truly bring a smile to your face. Is it playing with the children when you don't have something pressing waiting for you in the wings, or taking them to the local library for the Children's Story Hour? Is it going to visit friends, collecting rocks along the seashore or luxuriating in a bath, having a facial, then curling up with a good book? Maybe it's going skiing or to a movie or working on your favourite hobby; I spend my weekends trying to write a novel and believe me it can be very trying. You probably have very little time for these things that bring a smile to your face. So, consider your options and I hope this book will help you break the cycle.

Enough said, it's your choice!

One thing is for sure, that unless you win the Lottery, you will have to clean your place this week, next week and the next..... There's always going to be death, taxes and dust bunnies.

Chapter
THREE

CLEAN VS. TIDY

Chapter
THREE

Okay! Let's get to the subject of the book. How to maintain a *clean* home in just 2 hours a week! I will clarify the word *clean* later in this chapter. You know of course that my system works on a two-bedroom condominium. That's my place. This same system will also work for any three-bedroom house, apartment or condominium. If your home is a large two-story penthouse apartment or two-story four bedroom with finished basement house, resign yourself to probably a three-hour cleaning for you or anyone you hire. If you are in the practice of hiring help to clean your home, then establishing this schedule for them to follow will maintain a clean home and cost you less because of fewer hours of work.

We all have different standards. What is important to me may not be important to you. Conversely, you may have priorities in cleaning that would be on the bottom of my list. The schedule is yours to prepare and implement; I will simply guide you through the process.

For those of you who have been cleaning for many years, I am not trying to insult your abilities by telling you how to clean. My intent is to enlighten those people who have never had the guidance necessary to effectively clean. What I write is not cast in stone. (I would prefer it to be cast in gold anyway.) Make adjustments as you see fit. My basic idea is good, but everything can be improved upon, so use your own skills and judgments along the way to fulfill your personal needs.

At this point, I would like to clarify the misconception that I like cleaning. I don't hate cleaning, but I certainly don't like cleaning. It's just one of those chores that never goes away. It is there week after week after week. I do, however, think about my cleaning in a positive light. I'm always going to be cleaning, probably for the rest of my life, so why would I want to have the cleaning generate negative thoughts, which make the job harder. I must say though, since I established my **RCS**, it's so easy, I get upset if I actually have the nerve to complain to myself. Yes, to myself! I don't have anyone else who would listen to my complaints.

In the next chapter you will start the process, so I must establish one major point at this time.

When I use the word *clean*, I mean clean, not tidy. At no time does my system include or refer to tidying. If someone asked me to clean their place, I wouldn't hesitate. Well...maybe a little. If they asked me to tidy their place, I'd run a mile in the opposite direction. I've seen places that would take longer to tidy than to clean. I don't know why anyone would want to create such a workload. Of all the places I clean, only one is tidy when I arrive. It's a treat to do the cleaning and it makes the job so much easier. If your household is an untidy one, (*I know you're not the one who makes the mess only the one who cleans the mess*) you should consider tidying the night before. You could also consider using any method you see fit, short of impending death, to coerce the offenders into doing their own tidying. They tidy - You clean! Tidying while you clean lengthens the process and that's the last thing you need.

My old rather large Webster's Dictionary containing 2129 pages, gives the following definitions:

Clean: clear of dirt or filth; having all the uncleanness removed.
Tidy: neat in arrangement, in order.

I like the term, "having all the uncleanness removed". I immediately fantasized when I read that phrase. I would hire someone to clean my place, and then give instructions to "have all the uncleanness removed". *Can you imagine?* Then leave the house for a glorious carefree day. What a delicious thought, or more exact, dream!

I have never minded an untidy house. Having said this, I know that when my family reads this statement, they will say, Mother! They call me Mother when I upset them. It only takes one word with the right inflection. "Mother!" *Sound familiar?* What that means is, "Mom, you know that's not true." Well, I'm here to tell you, that it is true. You see I've never been able to convince anyone that the statement is true, perhaps, because the untidy house that I don't mind...is somebody else's house.

My friend Kathy came over for dinner last Sunday. She walked into my Condo and said, "Jean, your place is so....so....clean! It's just lovely." Hence, the book title.

In a matter-of-fact tone, I smugly replied, "I haven't done anything since Friday when I did my usual 2 hour cleaning." I know that sounded really smug. I sometimes forget how really clean my place looks. I exert such a small amount of energy to maintain this look that I'm still amazed at people's comments and if you adopt my **RCS**, people will make comments about your home. Very favourable comments! Your friends will be the first to notice.

Oh....by the way, I talked to my friend Kathy again. In the interest of the book, she is going to give my **RCS** a try.

So, here's wishing "happy times", "less trauma", and "saved hours", to all of you who will turn the page to find the real work!

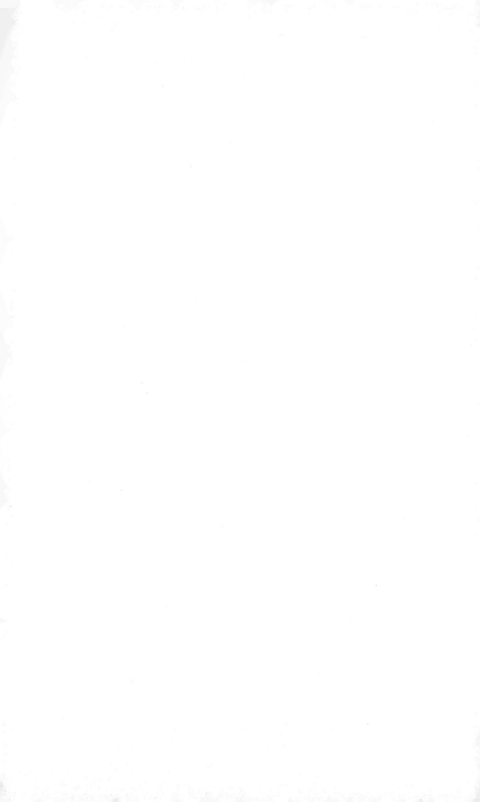

Chapter
FOUR

THE FIRST STEP

Chapter
FOUR

The purpose of this book is, a clean home, a clean home in fewer hours. It is my intention to save you time and allow you some freedom from this laborious task.

Do not be confused by the fact that you may only spend 2 hours now to clean your home. Do you remove all the *uncleanness*? This system will remove all the uncleanness forever. Your place will always have that extra glow, that sparkle and shine, that extra something that makes you feel proud.

If you don't think you should spend 2 hours a week cleaning, then I leave you with these thoughts:

- You will never again have to do that dreaded spring-cleaning!
- You will never scurry to do last minute cleaning when company is arriving with less than an hour's notice.
- You clean anyway. Why not spend the time doing the most effective and efficient job?
- You have an investment to protect! If you own your home, you have a valued property to keep intact. If you rent, you want two things: a recommendation when you move, plus your security deposit returned.

Whatever the reason, let's get to the first step.

The First Step must be completed before your **RCS** can be prepared.

The First Step

YOU MUST CLEAN EVERYTHING! I mean everything. Every baseboard, windowsill & ledge, mirrors, lamp shades, knick knacks, artificial floral arrangement, door frames, ceiling light fixtures, light bulbs (I'll explain later), EVERYTHING. Don't forget the stove, including the oven and refrigerator. Get the picture. Oh yes, don't forget the pictures.

Sound like a big job? Depending on your place, it may be an absolutely enormous, stupendous, immense, titanic, monstrous job. The saving grace, is you only have to do this job once. Adhere to the schedule that you will subsequently prepare and you will never again have to do a major cleaning. Certainly, 'spring cleaning' will take on a new name.

I have completed this first step on all but one of the units that I clean. Which unit didn't require the first step? You're right, the same one that's always tidy. This step has taken me from 4 hours to 8 hours to complete. The eight-hour job was in a large penthouse unit. The owners of this unit are slobs. This word is not my word. The lady of the house used these precise words, "we're slobs", on the day I accepted the cleaning position. I spend 6 hours every two weeks cleaning this unit and don't even come close to having all the uncleanness removed. Cleaning every two weeks is not sufficient to remove and control the dust in any home. This unit is my nemesis.

Here are some suggestions for the First Step;

a)   **If you're on your own,** prepare a pail of hot water with disinfectant and head towards the bathroom. In other words, **get started** and it will soon be over. You are definitely on your own.

b)   **If you are single, but share a residence,** then this is the ideal situation for my **RCS**. Assuming that you take turns with the cleaning, this is tailor-made for your place. Pick a time frame when you will all be home at the same time and share in the rigours of this First Step. When you're finished and while you're having a glass of wine or a slice of pizza (however you decide to reward yourself for a job well done) you can start work on your **RCS**. The most important factor to discuss at this time, while the aches and pains are still fresh, is who will bear the brunt of repeating the First Step if any individual does not complete their weeks cleaning exactly as per the schedule.

I can't repeat this often enough. You must adhere strictly to the schedule, each and every week.

c)   **Do you have children in the home?** Enlist their help. You and I both know they are the real creators of the dirt. You will have to find your own form of reason or a bribe unique to your situation.

Bottom line for them a parent who will now only have to spend two hours a week to maintain a clean home. (Remember, I said clean, not tidy) I'm sure they can understand your improved temperament when the cleaning is no longer drudgery. You simply have to accomplish the First Step. *Will they Help?* If, not, revert to suggestion **"a"**. You're on your own.

Speaking of children I am reminded of an incident, which you may find amusing. A number of years ago I called home on a Friday knowing my children would be home from school. I was calling to request they clean the house for me, as I would be working late. Unfortunately, my youngest daughter was the only one home. I proceeded to make my request anyway. I was pleased when she didn't hesitate and I looked forward to arriving home later that evening. At least until I got there! On first glance everything looked clean, but then I walked down the hall towards the bedrooms.

Raising my voice, I said, "You didn't do the bedrooms!"

Her quiet calm retort echoed down the hall, "I don't do bedrooms!"

Whenever I hear someone say they "don't do windows", I am reminded of this story. I do hope you have more success with your children.

e)   **Do you fall into the category of my friend Kathy?** It's Saturday afternoon and Kathy has just informed me that she will clean a room tonight. When she says a room, she does mean one room, then, maybe another room tomorrow and perhaps a room tomorrow evening. Of course, she still has the oven to clean. I told her to take as many days and evenings as she likes, as long as the schedule is prepared 7 days from the start of cleaning. The same goes for you. I wouldn't suggest taking 7 days for the First Step, because it will be time for your weekly 2 hour cleaning, before you're ready.

You are going to be exhausted when you are finished this major cleaning. You will not want to repeat this step in the near future, so I caution you again. You must make the commitment to complete each week's schedule, which you will soon prepare. You must commit to two-hours a week in order to always have a clean home.

For those who really hate cleaning, asking you to undertake this enormous task will seem somewhat akin to "walking the plank". The only words of wisdom I can impart would be to 'hire a maid service to remove all the uncleanness. If you decide to follow this suggestion you will have to be very specific in your instructions to the maid service. Some are not known for cleaning anything other than surfaces.

I make the foregoing suggestion based on my recent conversation with my friend Kathy.

I checked in with Kathy after a week, hoping she was preparing her schedule. Her cleaning wasn't complete. The reason went something like this, "I couldn't get involved with the cleaning; I was waiting for a phone call from....." Far be it for me to interfere with a new romance.

Another week passed and I called again, "No, I haven't finished the cleaning, but I've been thinking about it."

"This is good," I say. "Thinking about it, is good."

With all the times I've heard Kathy say she hates cleaning and the past week's procrastinations, I know it would take a small miracle for Kathy to ever undertake this intense cleaning.

Oh yes, her intentions are good and she really does want a clean place. There is just this over-riding unwillingness to enter into something so distasteful as a major cleaning.

I realize that some of you may feel the same way, hence, the suggestion of the maid service! Given the option, Kathy would hire someone to clean, but financially this is not something she can consider. The only way her schedule can be prepared is to have the First Step completed. So, in a couple of weeks I am going over to Kathy's place and will do her major cleaning. She is not crazy about the idea either, but I have insisted and will not take no for an answer. She must be a good friend.

You probably think I'm nuts and maybe I am, but I will never again have to listen to, "My place is so dirty." "My oven is so dirty." "It will probably take me all weekend to clean." ....*By the way! I am not cleaning the oven!!*

Remember, the result for your efforts in completing this First Step is only 2 hours of cleaning a week for a **So....So.... Clean!** home.

You may want to read the cleaning tips found in Chapter Ten before you start this First Step.

For the really uninitiated turn to the Addendum at the back of the book where I have detailed the cleaning in the First Step at Kathy's place.

Chapter
FIVE

PREPARING
THE SCHEDULE

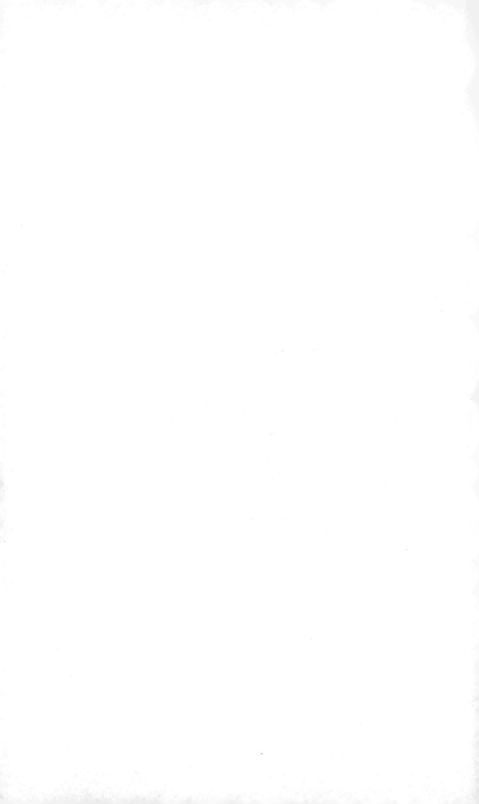

Chapter
FIVE

Is all the "uncleanness" removed? You are probably exhausted, but feel great. It's probably been a long time since your place looked quite this good. Stand back and take a good look around. You really must feel good. It was a big job and the best is yet to come. From this time forward your home will always look and be this clean. Now remember, I'm not talking about tidy or untidy, I'm talking about clean.

To prepare you for the philosophy of the system, I will tell you what does not go on the schedule. Normal dusting or vacuuming! Do not add to the schedule any item that must be cleaned every week. DON'T GET WORRIED THESE CHORES **ARE** INCLUDED IN THE 2 HOUR CLEANING TIME. You do not have to be reminded of what you clean each week. The schedule is designed to keep track of those items that will be cleaned on a bi-weekly or monthly or bi-monthly basis.

The schedule is to help you efficiently rotate those items that will not be cleaned weekly. For example, you will not add to your schedule the bathroom that you clean each week. Although, when you clean your bathroom you do not have to clean the light fixtures or shelf units or artificial flower arrangement. In order to keep your bathroom sparkling, you must clean these items, but not every week. So, the items that go on the schedule would be the bathroom light fixtures, the bathroom shelf unit, the flower arrangement and whatever extras your bathroom contains. As you will see in subsequent chapters, these items will sustain a clean look for six or more weeks.

Other items that require weekly cleaning and will not be added to the schedule are: normal dusting of your coffee and end tables, television, dresser, night tables etc., also the main vacuuming of visible areas. The areas behind your furniture and under the stereo etc. will go on the schedule and will not be a part of the weekly cleaning. You will not add to your schedule, the kitchen. You will add to your schedule the top of the refrigerator and the cupboard doors, which will become part of the remove fingerprints item that is placed on your schedule. Cleaning the top of the refrigerator does not mean we are neat freaks or perfectionists. We are simply removing any dust or dirt particles that could unsuspectingly take flight and land in the middle of your beautifully polished mahogany end table. This flight would probably happen as you opened the door to welcome your guests. To a small insignificant piece of dust, the opening of a door creates a veritable tornado, whirling through the rooms lifting all the hidden dust in its path and depositing it on all those beautifully gleaming surfaces.

You don't believe me? How many times have you cleaned your place for company and been perfectly satisfied with the look until you are sitting, quietly engrossed in conversation and your eyes spot a fine film of dust on that once clean end table. Cleaning places like the top of the refrigerator is what keeps a build-up of dust from covering your furniture during the week. Now that you know why we clean places that are out of sight, we are ready to continue.

The First Step, which you recently accomplished, has removed the majority of the dust. However, there is still dust in the air that will settle on your surfaces. As each cleaning week progresses through the schedule, your place will look better and better as you get rid of these dust particles. Dust particles are carried into the house on our hair, clothes, shoes, groceries, briefcases etc., but unless you have an army of people parading through your doors, this dust will not have much impact. If you do have a great deal of activity in your home, it will almost be impossible to achieve that extra glow. Your dust is continually taking flight then landing, taking flight and then landing. It's busier than the runways at La Guardia Airport! Trying to keep up with the dust is a hopeless cause, but with my system you should definitely achieve a brighter look.

Continuing with this same thought process, you probably will dust all your furniture surfaces when you clean, yet will seldom or never clean the baseboards. Did you know that your baseboards are the most dust-laden items in your home? Think about it. Whether it's carpet fibers or dust particles, we raise this dirt from the floor surfaces every time we move. Now, I'm not suggesting you do **the goose step.** As I know, when you walk through your rooms, you usually keep your feet fairly low to the floor and at the same time, keep the dust low. So, where do the dust and carpet fibers go that we raised from the floor? If not back on the floor surfaces, you'll find them on the baseboards. As I've said, the baseboards are one of the dirtiest items in your home. Now some of you may say, *So what?* I'll tell you what! If you are the type of person who likes to keep the furniture relatively dust-free or you are a surface cleaner, then you will only accomplish this by removing the dust culprits. Dust is what puts a dull finish over everything.

You can dust your furniture every day and if there is dust on your baseboards, it will be back on the furniture tomorrow, which is why you may find yourself in the position of having to dust daily.

Your schedule will consist of items that will be done on a rotating basis. Some items will be cleaned every second week, every third week, fourth etc. This process will become clearer as the chapter progresses.

Okay!....So one of the major items which must be cleaned on a scheduled basis are the baseboards. In fact, your baseboards will be cleaned every second week, as shown at the end of this chapter in **Exhibit #5-1**. If you look at this example, you will see that you are cleaning baseboards every week, but individual rooms are being cleaned on alternate weeks. Meaning, as I've stated, individual baseboards will be cleaned every second week.

Now that everything is clean, *I hope you cleaned the baseboards*, it is time to grab a piece of paper and lay out your schedule. It is easiest to do this directly following the First Step cleaning. All the items that require your total attention will be fresh in your mind.

At this point you will not know how many weeks your rotating schedule will span, so start as I have with 6 weeks. Most of the units I clean are on an 8 week schedule. The reason is not because their places are bigger that mine, it's because they have more paraphernalia to clean. As you will see, it is necessary to extend the schedule when your place contains a lot of extras.

To get started I have shown four examples at the end of this

Chapter. All exhibits within the book have been numbered with the first number denoting the chapter.

Exhibit # 5-1, assumes a one-level residence.

Exhibit # 5-2, assumes a one-level residence with finished basement.

Exhibit # 5-3, assumes a two-level residence.

Exhibit # 5-4, assumes a two-storey residence with finished basement.

I am not intentionally omitting anybody's residence layout in the Exhibits. If you have a split-level home you will probably rotate your baseboard cleaning on a 3 week rotational basis. You still have the same number of bedrooms as the one and two level residences, but you have more levels, therefore creating the third week rotation as in **Exhibits # 5-2** and **# 5-4**.

If you have a main level family room, because of the activity in this room, you will have to give it a separate slot on the schedule.

So that you can get an initial feel for the completed schedule, I have included two additional examples at the end of this chapter.

Exhibit # 5-5, is a 1300 square foot unit that I clean. This is an 8 week **RCS**. The reason for the extended schedule is the number of artificial flower arrangements in this residence and the kitchen chairs and dining room table slotted in Weeks 5 and 6. The kitchen chairs are black lacquer that require a good cleaning to remove oily fingerprints. The dining room table is bamboo and has a center post with five splayed legs. The design of this table creates many hiding places for the dust; therefore, I have given the table its own time

Exhibit # 5-6, is a 1600 square foot unit, also one of my regular cleaning jobs. This schedule spans 9 weeks. This is a penthouse unit and has many areas of glass and mirrors. In addition to this, the unit has three chesterfields and two large bookcases. You will notice that the bookcase in the family room has been placed on the schedule twice during the 9 week **RCS**, but the guest room bookcase only once, as this room does not have as much activity. Another item to note is the silver in Weeks 4 and 5. The silver that I polish in these weeks are, candlesticks, salt and pepper shakers, butter dish, candy dish, two vases and a five-rack collection of spoons. All these items are on display. When's the last time you cleaned your silver? Just before that once a year visit from the mother-in-law or worse, your mother! *I jest!* I will admit that these two particular weeks add an additional 5 minutes to the schedule, but time well spent.

In reviewing these Exhibits I'm sure it did not miss your attention that I included the windowsills with the baseboards. As the ledges must be cleaned, I have found it efficient to clean them at the same time as the baseboards. You may find that your windowsills can be included when you remove fingerprints.

In this chapter I have given four examples to enable you to start your own schedule. However, in future chapters, for clarity, I will be using the **RCS** in **Exhibit # 5-1**. When slotting your baseboards don't be too concerned that you may be cleaning them less often than every second week.

Although every second week is ideal, you can still achieve the same results with an extended schedule. It will just take a little longer to get the dust under control. Eventually you will have friends say, "Your place is **So...So...Clean**!"

The part of this method I like the best is the time saving. In 2 or 3 minutes I can clean the baseboards and windows areas in most rooms. When I have to move heavy furniture, it will take me a good 5 minutes. The other advantage to this method is, while you are down on all fours it is very easy to wipe under some of the furniture that is too heavy to move and where the vacuum doesn't reach. Also, wipe the base of furniture that is at floor level.

At one time I used my dusting attachment to vacuum my baseboards and windowsills. I would then remove the attachment and use the nozzle to vacuum the junction of the carpet and baseboards, an area famous for dust build-up, as the floor or carpet attachments are not designed to reach this crevice. *We can guess who designs vacuum cleaners!* For many years I thought this to be a most effective method. Since I have been in the position of using different vacuums and some of those being upright models as opposed to my canister type, I've had to resort to another method of cleaning these areas, by hand. So, I prepared a pail of hot water with a drop of disinfectant cleaner (too much will leave streaks, depending on the surface) and with little aplomb, got down on my hands and knees and wiped the base-boards, the carpet junction and the windowsills along with other ledges on the window or heat registers. Much to my surprise, this method is not only faster, but also definitely more effective in eliminating the dust.

Just before we leave this slot on the schedule, I will tell you that this is a 15-minute time slot, 3 or 5 minutes for each room. If you look again at **Exhibit # 5-1**, Weeks 1, 3 and 5 will take 15 minutes only if you have three bedrooms. Weeks 2, 4 and 6 are definitely 15 minutes, as you will probably be moving furniture. No! I don't think you are a female version of Arnold Schwarzenager, just an ordinary house frau who over the years has proven she can do most anything.

EXHIBIT # 5-1

RCS FOR A ONE-LEVEL RESIDENCE

Week 1 - Baseboards & Windowsills, Bedrooms & Hallways

Week 2 - Baseboards & Windowsills, Living & Dining Rooms & Kitchen

Week 3 - Baseboards & Windowsills, Bedrooms & Hallways

Week 4 - Baseboards & Windowsills, Living & Dining Rooms & Kitchen

Week 5 - Baseboards & Windowsills, Bedrooms & Hallways

Week 6 - Baseboards & Windowsills, Living & Dining Rooms & Kitchen

EXHIBIT # 5-2

RCS FOR A ONE-LEVEL RESIDENCE WITH FINISHED BASEMENT

Week 1 - Baseboards & Windowsills, Bedrooms & Hallways

-
-
-
-

Week 2 - Baseboards & Windowsills, Living & Dining Rooms & Kitchen

-
-
-
-

Week 3 - Baseboards & Windowsills, Finished Basement

-
-
-
-

Week 4 - Baseboards & Windowsills, Bedrooms & Hallways

-
-
-
-

Week 5 - Baseboards & Windowsills, Living & Dining Rooms & Kitchen

-
-
-
-

Week 6 - Baseboards & Windowsills, Finished Basement

-
-
-
-

EXHIBIT # 5-3

RCS FOR A TWO-LEVEL RESIDENCE

Week 1 - Baseboards & Windowsills, Upstairs
-
-
-
-

Week 2 - Baseboards & Windowsills, Downstairs
-
-
-
-

Week 3 - Baseboards & Windowsills, Upstairs
-
-
-
-

Week 4 - Baseboards & Windowsills, Downstairs
-
-
-
-

Week 5 - Baseboards & Windowsills, Upstairs
-
-
-
-

Week 6 - Baseboards & Windowsills, Downstairs
-
-
-
-

EXHIBIT # 5-4

RCS FOR A TWO-LEVEL RESIDENCE WITH FINISHED BASEMENT

Week 1 - Baseboards & Windowsills, Upstairs
-
-
-
-

Week 2 - Baseboards & Windowsills, Downstairs
-
-
-
-

Week 3 - Baseboards & Windowsills, Finished Basement
-
-
-
-

Week 4 - Baseboards & Windowsills, Upstairs
-
-
-
-

Week 5 - Baseboards & Windowsills, Downstairs
-
-
-
-

Week 6 - Baseboards & Windowsills, Finished Basement
-
-
-
-

EXHIBIT #5-5

A 1300 SQUARE FOOT UNIT - COMPLETED RCS

Week 1 - B & W, Bedrooms & Hallways
- Mirrored Closet Doors, Bedrooms & Foyer
- Chesterfields
- Lights Master Bedroom & Ceiling Fan
- Wax Bedroom Floor

Week 2 - B & W Living/Dining Rooms & Kitchen
- French Doors
- Lamps
- Washer/Dryer
- A.F.A.

Week 3 - B & W, Bedrooms & Hallways
- Mirrored Closet Doors, Bedrooms & Foyer
- Tub Mirrors
- Top of Refrigerator
- Fingerprints

Week 4 - B & W Living/Dining Rooms & Kitchen
- French Doors
- Pictures/Mirrors
- Stove & Exhaust Fan
- A.F.A.

Abbreviations

A.F.A.- Artificial Flower Arrangements
B & W - Baseboards & Windowsills

Week 5 - B & W, Bedrooms & Hallways
- Mirrored Closet Doors, Bedrooms & Foyer
- Bathroom Bar Lights
- Kitchen Chairs
- Wax Hallway

Week 6 - Mirrored Closet Doors, Bedrooms & Foyer
- French Doors
- Walk-in-Closet
- Dining Room Table
- A.F.A.

Week 7 - B & W, Bedrooms & Hallways
- Mirrored Closet Doors, Bedrooms & Foyer
- Ceiling Light Fixtures
- Tub Mirrors
- Dresser

Week 8 - B & W Living/Dining Rooms & Kitchen
- French Doors
- Doors & Doorframes
- Move Stove & Refrigerator
- A.F.A.

EXHIBIT #5-6

A 1600 SQUARE FOOT UNIT - COMPLETED RCS

Week 1 - B & W, Bedrooms & Hallways
- Mirrored Closet Doors, Bedrooms & Foyer
  - Spice Rack
- Stereo Unit

Week 2 - B & W Living/Dining Rooms & Kitchen
- Mirrored Foyer Closet Living Room
  - Bathroom Bar Lights
  - Bookcase Family Room
  - A.F.A.

Week 3 - B $& W Solarium
  - French Doors
  - Curio Cabinet
  - Tea Wagon
  - Fingerprints

Week 4 - B & W, Bedrooms & Hallways
- Mirrored Closet Doors, Bedrooms & Foyer
  - Chesterfields
  - Bookcase Guest Room
  - Silver

Week 5 - B & W, Living/Dining Rooms & Kitchen
- Mirrored Foyer Closet Living Room
  - Fireplace & Mantle
  - Buffet
  - Silver

Week 6 - B & W, Solarium
  - French Doors
  - Solarium Doors
  - Move Wine Rack
  - A.F.A.

Week 7 - B & W, Bedrooms & Hallways
- Mirrored Closet Doors, Bedrooms & Foyer
  - Solarium Doors
  - Bookcase, Family Room
  - Doors & Doorframes

Week 8 - B & W Living/Dining Rooms & Kitchen
- Mirrored Foyer Closet Living Room
  - Chesterfields
  - Guest Room Ensuite Bathroom Lights
  - A.F.A.

Week 9 - B & W , Solarium
  - French Doors
  - Solarium
  - Washer/Druer
  - Computer Unit

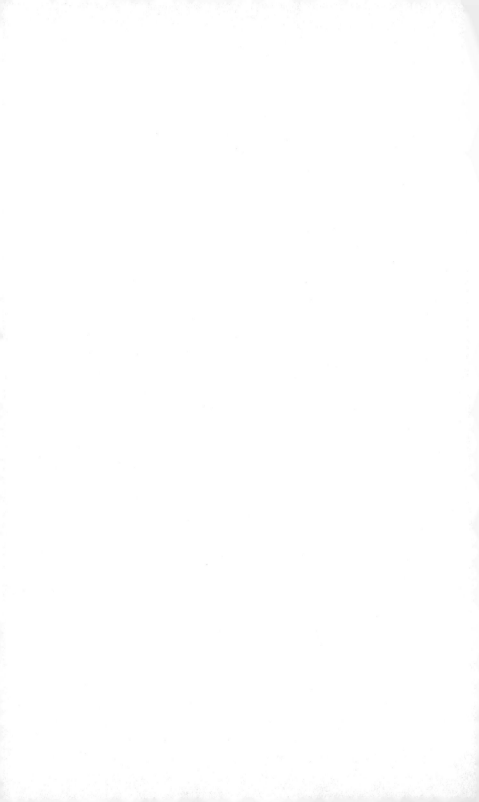

Chapter
SIX

FIFTEEN MINUTE JOBS

Chapter
SIX

The schedule you are preparing covers a time period of 45 minutes. Let me tell you at this time that the regular cleaning, which does not go on the schedule, takes approximately 1 hour and 15 minutes: for some people a little less and for others a little more time, but these will be the exceptions.

The regular cleaning is the once over, fast, surface cleaning you always do when company is coming. You clean your bathrooms, then run through the place wiping every visible surface, then grab the vacuum cleaner and go over the major carpet areas. I know I used to do the same thing. You can probably accomplish this in 1 hour flat, because you've had lots of practice. Remember, you will never have to do this last minute cleaning again. Your place will always look presentable and clean. The only last minute thing you may want to do will be a little tidying. Think about it. Company can arrive unexpectedly anytime and you will never again be traumatized by a place that you just haven't had the time to clean.

The 45 minute **RCS** you will prepare for each week to complete the two-hour cleaning is comprised of 2, 15-minute time slots and 3, 5-minute time slots.

The baseboards and windowsills, as previously mentioned and which you have placed in the first position, are a 15-minute job. This item will be something that your standards may deem a priority. You may place this item on the schedule every week or bi-weekly depending on the necessity of the job or the number of items in your place that require 15 minute time slots.

Other items that could qualify for the second 15-minute time slot are shown in **Exhibit #6-1** at the end of this chapter:

Fingerprints on Walls and Doorframes

If you have children in the home you probably clean fingerprints every day and never have the job finished. Although you may clean these on a daily basis, it would still be a good idea to have them on your schedule, so that you can take the time to thoroughly clean these areas. These places would be added in the second position, possibly bi-weekly. *I wonder in which century they will invent ever so thin rays of ultra violet beams next to our walls that could gently 'zap' the would be offenders.*

Sliding Glass Doors

One of the places I clean has double French doors in three locations a 15 minute job and another place has large triple glass door in two locations adjoining the solarium, another 15 minute job.

Mirrored Closet Doors

This is my item. I have triple sliding mirrored doors in both bedrooms and the foyer, as well as glass doors adjoining the solarium. I personally love clean mirrors, so I do this job as often as possible. See **Exhibit # 6-1**, position 2, at the end of this chapter.

Large Stereo Cabinets, Bookcases or Wall/Computer Units

These are very visible items and if you are fortunate enough to add them to a 15 minute time slot on the schedule, then you will have the necessary time it takes to clean them thoroughly and always have them looking clean. Otherwise, you will be relegated to cleaning this during the regular portion of the cleaning and be rushed in the process. Just a note. The place I clean that I call my nemesis, takes me 15 minutes to clean the top of the bedroom dresser. I will let your imagination picture how it must look.

If you do not have items such as I have mentioned that will fill a 15-minute time slot, then follow this criteria. Find two or three items, which take 5 minutes each to clean and slot them in the second 15-minute position.

You could consider putting your oven, (*ooh...that four letter word*), in this time slot. Most of us cannot put our oven on the schedule and must clean it at a completely different time. I don't have a problem here. Much to Kathy's chagrin, I have a self cleaning oven.

You may add your refrigerator. That item we never quite seem to get around to cleaning or, perhaps I shouldn't assume. I don't get around to cleaning it. I am not able to add this item to my schedule and it definitely is a 15 minute job. I am cursed with a poorly designed kitchen. You know the type I mean! The kitchens that men design for us! My apologies to all the men reading this book as my statement is made from generalized precedents. In somebody's wisdom, they placed a left-hand opening refrigerator next to a right-hand wall in my kitchen. The door to my refrigerator will not open greater than to a perpendicular position before it hits the wall and I am unable to remove my vegetable and meat trays. I have tried wriggling my nose with my finger, "Door be gone". I've never had much success with this avenue of thinking, so I then must revert to reality. I must pull the refrigerator into the middle of the floor. Considering the closequarters in which most of these units are placed, I'm sure you know this requires a back and forth pulling motion as it slowly inches forward . Now the refrigerator is clear of it's space, but the side is still flush with the wall. I must then angle the refrigerator to the center of the kitchen before I can open the door sufficiently to remove the trays and clean. Do I clean my refrigerator often? No! Am I pleased with the designers of the kitchen? No! I have never been pleased with the design of any kitchen. In one of my daughters' kitchen, her refrigerator door bangs into a cupboard, which is perpendicular to the refrigerator wall. *Lord have mercy! Who designs kitchens?*

Perhaps your busy schedule doesn't allow you to wipe your cupboards at meal times. Your cupboards would then be a perfect item for this 15-minute time slot. This time would give you the opportunity to not only wipe the face of the cupboards, but to clean the inside of the doors and clean the inside of your condiment cupboard and the cupboard under the sink and your silverware drawer. (And you would have time left over.) If this sounds like things are getting just a little out of hand, work with me on this, you're still only cleaning two hours a week.

Although these items may currently take you more than 15 minutes to clean, when they are added to the schedule and cleaned on a regular basis, they will only take you 15 minutes or less to clean. The little amount of time required to clean most items is created by the **RCS**, which never allows for a build-up of dirt. I can't see inside your home, remember wriggling my nose doesn't work. Nor can I foresee your priorities, so selecting this item will require some thought on your part.

If you select only one item, then you can clean this item each week. If you select two items, then you can alternate these on a bi-weekly basis. If you select three items, then you can slot them alternately over the 6 weeks. This means, one item would be cleaned once every 3 weeks or twice in the 6 weeks schedule.

I do understand in advance that some of you may have six or more 15 minute items. This of course means that once every 6 weeks, one of your items will get cleaned or in the case of eight items you must go to an 8 week schedule and those items would only get cleaned once in 8 weeks. If you fall into this category, I'm sure that these items are not currently being cleaned as often as you would like and I hope this schedule will help lift and lighten this burden. You may not achieve that **So.... So.... Clean!** look, but you will be pleased that your cleaning is under control and your place certainly does look and feel brighter.

I'm sure you've guessed, that one of my friend Kathy's 15 minute items is, **the infamous oven**! Be like Kathy. Find those items you hate to do and place them on the schedule. Believe me, they will no longer become a burden. Spend 15 minutes or less once a week for one of these items and it will never prey on your mind again.

The schedule is not complicated, but as I've said, it does take considerable thought on your part so that you will be able to go to your 2 hour weekly **RCS** each week and not have to think about it the rest of the week. Instead you can think about brownies (for some it's the edible variety), baseball practice and helping with the dreaded math homework and so on. (If only you had paid attention in math class....HELP! It's terrible when your kids get smarter than you.)

EXHIBIT # 6-1

RCS FOR A ONE-LEVEL RESIDENCE

Week 1 - Baseboards & Windowsills, Upstairs
- Mirrored Closet Doors, Bedrooms & Foyer
-
-

Week 2 - Baseboards & Windowsills, Downstairs
- Mirrored Closet Doors, Foyer & Glass Doors Solarium
-
-

Week 3 - Baseboards & Windowsills, Finished Basement
- Mirrored Closet Doors, Bedrooms & Foyer
-
-

Week 4 - Baseboards & Windowsills, Upstairs
- Mirrored Closet Doors, Foyer & Glass Doors Solarium
-
-

Week 5 - Baseboards & Windowsills, Downstairs
- Mirrored Closet Doors, Bedrooms & Foyer
-
-

Week 6 - Baseboards & Windowsills, Finished Basement
- Mirrored Closet Doors, Foyer & Glass Doors Solarium
-
-

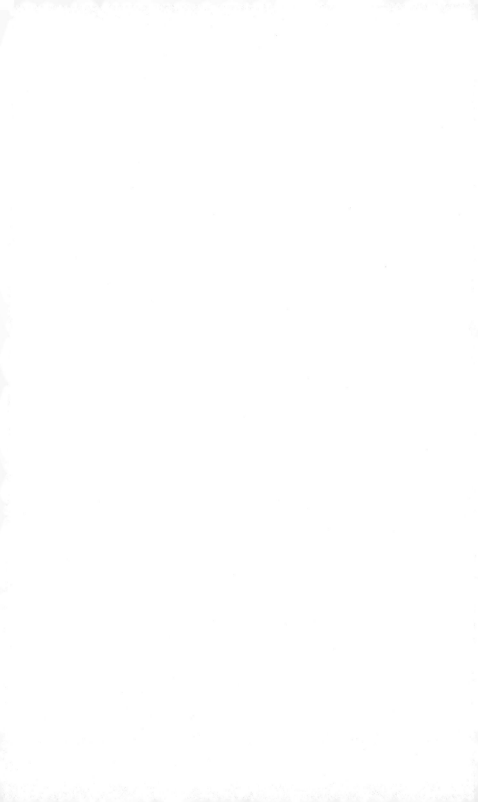

Chapter
SEVEN

FIVE MINUTE JOBS

Chapter
SEVEN

If you have completed filling the 15 minute slots on your schedule, then it is time for a final tour of your place. The remaining three items per week on the schedule will be comprised of 5 minute items. All the remaining items in your home should fall into this category.

You will need a separate piece of paper. Make a rough list of every remaining item in your home similar to my list.

Door Frames
Fingerprints
Chesterfield & Chairs
Lamps
Pictures
Ceiling Light Fixtures
Bathroom Mirror & Lights
Artificial Flower Arrangement
Top of Refrigerator
Shelf Unit
Top of Buffet
Inside Curio Cabinet
Bookcase
Tea Wagon
Fireplace
Spice Rack
Washer/Dryer
Stove Exhaust Fan

This list includes eighteen items. If your schedule follows mine and spans a 6 week period you can have up to eighteen items to be included on the remaining schedule. This will allow you to clean each item once every 6 weeks. If your list totals a greater number of items, then you will have to extend your schedule. Be careful when adding weeks.

Note that in Chapter 5, **Exhibit # 5-1** and **Exhibit # 5-3**, where areas are being cleaned on a bi-weekly basis, your schedule must have an even number of weeks. If your residence falls into these exhibits and you must extend the weeks, then your schedule would go from 6 weeks to 8 weeks. You must always have an even number of weeks. Of course, with everything, there is always exceptions. So, if they arise for you, go with it!

If your residence falls under **Exhibit # 5-2** or **Exhibit # 5-4**, where your areas are being cleaned every third week, then an extended schedule would include an additional three weeks. You would have a 9 week **RCS**, not the best, but workable. After all, Kathy's **RCS** is 10 weeks. (shown as **Exhibit # 11-1** at the end of Chapter Eleven.)

Let me explain the items on my list so that you will have a better understanding of why some items falling into this category may or may not fall into the regular cleaning that is not on the schedule. You really do not want to have these items included in your regular cleaning, which is not on the schedule. Let me remind you that the regular cleaning is the once over, quick to get done, cleaning. We don't want anything left to the regular cleaning that would not get the attention required to keep it in a clean state.

Door Frames - These are an easy 5 minute job and consists of taking a damp cloth and wiping down the doors including the top of the doors and doorframes. When the dust comes under control this item will stay clean for almost 8 weeks and will not be subject to taking flight.

Chesterfield & Chairs - These items include the vacuuming of all upholstered furniture. If you have animals or children and you don't have a total of eighteen items on your list, then you may want to consider putting this item down more that once every 6 weeks. If your units are leather then a damp cloth soaked with a disinfectant cleaner will do the job and then use your own care products to bring the leather, back to its supple nature.

Lamps - The lamps require vacuuming of the lampshade and cleaning the base. You are the best judge of how you clean your base whether it is glass, porcelain, brass, wood etc. There are so many variables that I leave this one up to you. Don't forget to wipe off the bulb with a damp cloth. I will cover this item in greater detail under 'ceiling light fixtures'.

Pictures - Pictures require a wiping of the frames; don't forget to reach behind the top of the frame (the dust bunnies think this is the best hiding place). In my place this is definitely a 5-minute item as I have forty-four pictures with twenty-six having a glass front.

Ceiling Light Fixtures - This is one of those items you may currently leave until spring-cleaning time, but remember, no more spring cleaning (except of course for window washing and cleaning the curtains or dry-cleaning drapes). You will use a damp cloth to wipe the shade and the bulbs. Yes, the bulbs! If you saw the movie Driving Miss Daisy, you will remember the scene where she asked her chauffeur what he was doing. Although it was quite evident that he was cleaning the bulbs in the chandelier, upon his response, "I'm cleaning the bulbs", her retort was, "Whoever heard of such a silly thing?" These may not be the exact words, but the scene brought a smile to my face, knowing that I clean my bulbs. The heat of the bulbs attracts dust particles and it is quite surprising how much more light will shine when the bulbs are clean. Everything is just that much brighter. Make sure the light is turned off and cool when you clean the bulb. This cleaning goes a long way in achieving that *So....So....Clean!'* look.

Bathroom Mirror & Lights - In my bathroom, I have mirrors that cover the wall from ceiling to counter. It is not necessary to clean the entire mirror when I clean the bathroom on a regular basis. So, I add this item to my list to be cleaned at the same time as the bathroom light fixtures. One of my bathrooms is easy, as the light fixtures consist of two lamps on each side of the mirror over the counter, but the other bathroom has a set of bar lights with ten bulbs on a metal rack, which also has to be polished. Can you believe that in a small bathroom someone decided that it needed the power of ten bulbs? This is overkill.

Artificial Flower Arrangements - Before I even explain how I clean my arrangements, I will acknowledge that a spray is available on the market and does an excellent job in just seconds. This is not my choice, so I set about with a damp cloth wiping each petal. Fortunately, I have only two, not like one of my cleaning units where they have an arrangement on every surface and on the floor in every corner. This is one of those items you may have left for spring-cleaning, but your control of the dust will be further advanced if you place this on your schedule for regular cleaning. By the way, I have twenty-three live plants and I have yet to figure out how they could be included on the schedule and still keep it to the 2 hours. I find a couple of hours once every 3 or 4 months and take care of this item. Don't worry about the dust taking flight while on the leaves. This doesn't happen. You just clean the leaves in order for the plant to breathe.

Top of Refrigerator - This is a nice and easy item and just another of those items that would never get done on a regular basis if not for the schedule. Add this item to the list on a week where you have a hard 5 minute job.

Shelf Unit - I added this item to my list, because every one has a shelf unit someplace. This can be one of those items you don't like doing because it requires taking everything off the shelf, wiping it, then wiping everything else before putting it back. As I clean several shelf units, I can promise you that the task seems much bigger than it actually is. I don't have one that takes me more than 5 minutes. It just seems like an onerous job. Don't move things around trying to clean under them, then sliding them back into place or it will be more than a 5 minute job. So, remove everything, wipe the shelf then return each item after it has been wiped.

Top of Buffet - In the course of your regular cleaning you quite naturally wipe down the buffet or dust the edges, but the last thing you want to do every week (nor is it necessary) is climb upon a chair and clean the top of the unit. That is why this item is best left to a 5 minute scheduled time slot. As this item does not take 5 minutes to clean, use your discretion as to filling this time slot. You could clean the glass door of the buffet or include more than one cabinet in this time slot to fill the 5 minutes.

Inside Curio Cabinet - As with the buffet, you will not clean inside the cabinet on a regular basis, but you will add this item to your schedule so that you can give the knick-knacks and shelves a good cleaning. After all, if you have a curio cabinet, it's there to show off your collection. So make sure it shines, especially for you and remember you will still be staying within the 2 hour **RCS**. This item definitely takes a full 5 minutes and later I will explain how to break down your list into 'hard' and 'easy' 5 minute jobs.

Bookcase - This is an item, which your own standards will have to establish how much cleaning you will complete. I normally remove all the books, wipe the shelf then put the books back. It still astounds me how much work you can accomplish in five minutes. Hard to believe, but this is only a five minute job.

Tea Wagon - When I put the tea wagon on my list it normally means to move it from the wall and clean the baseboards, then clean the wheels and the other areas that do not get cleaned during my regular cleaning. This too is another one of those items that can get left until you can't stand looking at the dust anymore.

Fireplace - I don't have a fireplace, but the penthouse unit I clean has a beautiful one with an intricate carved screen and all. When it is time to do this item I move the screen, then wipe the hearth area as well as the intricate design on the mantle face and the screen. I also have time to remove any ashes and vacuum the residue. I still complete the job within the 5 minutes.

Spice Rack - This item isall too often forgotten. We usually handle our spices when we are cooking and all too often have food on our hands. It really only takes 5 minutes to remove the bottles, wipe them down and replace them after wiping the shelf. So put this item on your schedule and you will be pleased when you walk into the kitchen and see your clean rack. Items like this will bring a smile to your face. You will be exerting so little effort to accomplish this task that you will feel delighted.

Washer/Dryer - This is an area which always has a great deal of lint and although you probably wipe away most of it when you're using the machines, I find it necessary to add this item to my list, so that I can really give the whole area a good cleaning.

Stove Exhaust Fan - This is a another forgotten item. Most stoves have an overhead fan where the filter can be removed and washed. Cleaning the fan on a regular basis will keep it more effective, preventing grease laden dust from circulating.

You must feel exhausted just reading all this information. I'm sure you find it hard to believe at this point that all these items can be completed and still stay within the 2 hour weekly schedule or you may be thinking that you can forget about half of the things because you don't care about them and you will save yourself even more time. Well, 15 minutes a week is not going to kill you and that's all the combined time required to complete the cleaning of these items. It's the combination of cleaning each and every item in your home along with the rotating schedule that keeps the dust under control and allows you to complete these tasks in such a short time frame. Remember, that the objective is to have a *So.... So.... Clean!*', home in just **Two Hours A Week** and you can accomplish that extra glow if you follow the course I am setting before you.

I think it's time to remind you of the unsuspecting dust that rises when least expected and lands on your beautifully polished surfaces. It's not the dust you can see that causes the problems; it's the dust particles you normally can't see that are the culprits. So, take the time while preparing your schedule to ensure that all those out-of-sight areas are going to get the attention they require.

Take the time now to segregate some of the items on your list. Divide the list into **Hard 5 Minute Jobs** and **Easy 5 Minute Jobs**. So, if you are staying with a 6 week schedule, you will not want more than six **Hard 5 Minute Jobs** and twelve **Easy 5 Minute Jobs** to fill the eighteen remaining slots. My list breaks down as follows;

Hard 5 Minute Jobs
Chesterfield & Chairs
Ceiling Light Fixtures
Shelf Unit
Inside Curio Cabinet
Bookcase
Spice Rack

Easy 5 Minute Jobs

Doors & Door Frames
Lamps
Pictures
Bathroom Mirror & Lights
Artificial Flower Arrangement, Dining Room Table
Artificial Flower Arrangement, Ensuite Bathroom
Top of Refrigerator
Top of Buffet
Tea Wagon
Fireplace
Washer/Dryer
Stove Exhaust

Now take your **Hard 5 Minute Jobs** and place them in the third position on your schedule. See **Exhibit # 7-1**.

A small caution at this time! The first position in Weeks 2, 4 and 6 are items that require a good 15 minutes work, since I move most of the furniture when doing this job. For this reason I try to put the 5 minute jobs requiring the least work in these positions. As an example, the *inside curio cabinet* item, that is a full 5 minutes work, has been placed in Week 3 and would not be a balanced workload if placed in either of Weeks 2, 4 or 6. Try to adjust your schedule to even the workload each week. You may have to go through the first complete rotation of the schedule before you are able to make the adjustments.

Preparing the schedule is a big job I know, but it's starting to take shape. If you've been sitting around having a glass of wine while preparing the schedule, you may be in good shape as well. *smiles*

EXHIBIT # 7-1

RCS FOR A ONE-LEVEL RESIDENCE

Week 1 - Baseboards & Windowsills, Bedroom & Hallways
- Mirrored Closet Doors, Bedrooms & Foyer
- Vacuum Chesterfield & Chairs
-
-

Week 2 - Baseboards & Windowsills, Living & Dining Rooms & Kitchen
- Mirrored Closet Doors, Foyer & Glass Doors Solarium
- Ceiling Light Fixtures
-
-

Week 3 - Baseboards & Windowsills, Bedroom & Hallways
- Mirrored Closet Doors, Bedrooms & Foyer
- Inside Curio Cabinet
-
-

Week 4 - Baseboards & Windowsills, Living & Dining Rooms & Kitchen
- Mirrored Closet Doors, Foyer & Glass Doors Solarium
- Shelf Unit Kitchen
-
-

Week 5 - Baseboards I Windowsills, Bedroom & Hallways
- Mirrored Closet Doors, Bedrooms & Foyer
- Bookcase
-
-

Week 6 - Baseboards & Windowsills, Living & Dining Rooms & Kitchen
- Mirrored Closet Doors, Foyer & Glass Doors Solarium
- Spice Rack
-
-

Chapter
EIGHT

EASY/VERY EASY

5 MINUTE JOBS

Chapter
EIGHT

We will now concern ourselves with re-defining the "Easy 5 Minute Jobs". Take a look at your remaining items and break them down into two separate groups. **Easy 5 Minute Jobs** and **Very Easy 5 Minute Jobs.** The **Very Easy 5 Minute Job**s will consist of those items, which we know will only take about 2 minutes to clean. Most of the items remaining on your list really do not consist of 5 minutes work, but I classify them as such in order to have breathing room. It gives you those extra few minutes to go to the refrigerator for a cold drink.

Yes, it's time for another piece of paper. Of the remaining twelve items, split them into two six item groups. If you are on a schedule longer than 6 weeks you will have more than twelve items, but use the same principle to divide them.

Easy 5 Minute Jobs

Door Frames
Bathroom Mirror & Light Fixtures
Tea Wagon
Fireplace
Washer/Dryer
Stove Exhaust Fan

These Easy 5 Minute Jobs will be placed in the fourth position on your schedule, as in **Exhibit # 8-1** at the end of this Chapter.

Very Easy 5 Minute Jobs

Lamps
Pictures
Artificial Flower Arrangements, Dining Room Table
Artificial Flower Arrangement, Ensuite Bathroom
Top of Refrigerator
Top of Buffet

These last six items will be added to the schedule in the fifth position, as shown in **Exhibit # 8-2**, at the end of this Chapter.

Spend the next 10 minutes reading the remainder of the book, then return to your schedule and try one last time to even out the workload with the individual weeks. Don't become too stressed with balancing the workload, the balance will become evident as you progress through the **Rotating Cleaning System**.

EXHIBIT # 8-1

RCS FOR A ONE-LEVEL RESIDENCE

Week 1 - Baseboards & Windowsills, Upstairs
   - Mirrored Closet Doors, Bedrooms & Foyer
   - Vacuum Chesterfield & Chairs
   - Door Frames
   -

Week 2 - Baseboards & Windowsills, Downstairs
   - Mirrored Closet Doors, Foyer & Glass Doors Solarium
   - Ceiling Light Fixtures
   - Washer Dryer
   -

Week 3 - Baseboards & Windowsills, Finished Basement
   - Mirrored Closet Doors, Bedrooms & Foyer
   - Inside Curio Cabinet
   - Bathroom Mirror & Light Fixtures
   -

Week 4 - Baseboards & Windowsills, Upstairs
   - Mirrored Closet Doors, Foyer & Glass Doors Solarium
   - Shelf Unit Kitchen
   - Stove Exhaust Fan
   -

Week 5 - Baseboards & Windowsills, Downstairs
   - Mirrored Closet Doors, Bedrooms & Foyer
   - Bookcase
   - Tea Wagon
   -

Week 6 - Baseboards & Windowsills, Finished Basement
   - Mirrored Closet Doors, Foyer & Glass Doors Solarium
   - Spice Rack
   - Fireplace
   -

EXHIBIT # 8-2

RCS FOR A ONE-LEVEL RESIDENCE

Week 1 - Baseboards & Windowsills, Bedrooms & Hallways
- Mirrored Closet Doors, Bedrooms & Foyer
- Vacuum Chesterfield & Chairs
- Door Frames
- Lamps

Week 2 - Baseboards & Windowsills, Living & Dining Rooms & Kitchen
- Mirrored Closet Doors, Foyer & Glass Doors Solarium
- Ceiling Light Fixtures
- Washer Dryer
- Top of Refrigerator

Week 3 - Baseboards & Windowsills, Bedrooms & Hallways
- Mirrored Closet Doors, Bedrooms & Foyer
- Inside Curio Cabinet
- Bathroom Mirror & Light Fixtures
- Artificial Flower Arrangement, Ensuite Bathroom

Week 4 - Baseboards & Windowsills, Living & Dining Rooms & Kitchen
- Mirrored Closet Doors, Foyer & Glass Doors Solarium
- Shelf Unit Kitchen
- Stove Exhaust Fan
- Artificial Flower Arrangements, Dining Room Table

Week 5 - Baseboards & Windowsills, Bedrooms & Hallways
- Mirrored Closet Doors, Bedrooms & Foyer
- Bookcase
- Tea Wagon
- Top of Buffet

Week 6 - Baseboards & Windowsills, Living & Dining Rooms & Kitchen
- Mirrored Closet Doors, Foyer & Glass Doors Solarium
- Spice Rack
- Fireplace
- Pictures

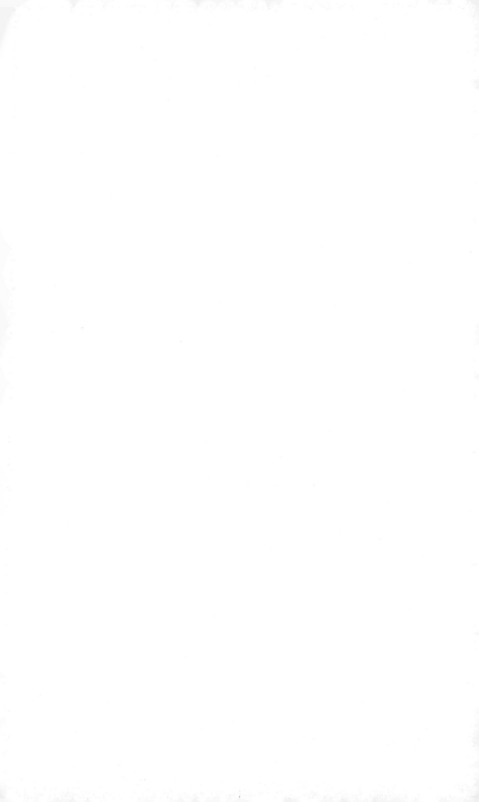

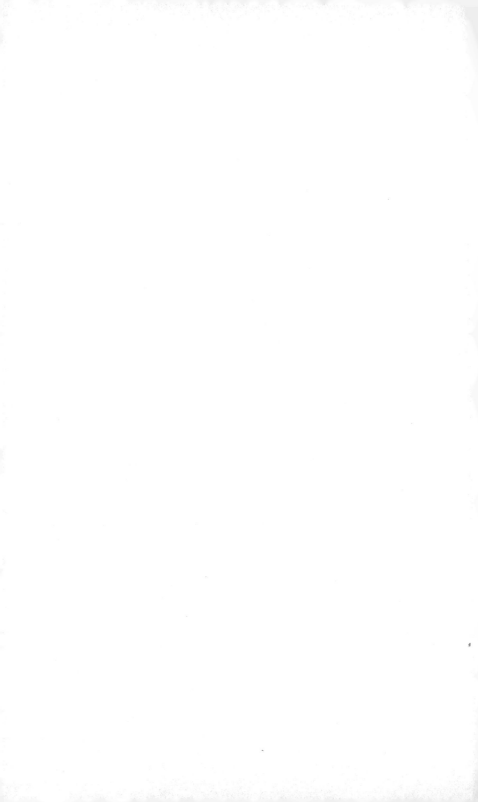

Chapter
NINE

THE 'HOW TO'
AND 'WHAT FOR'

Chapter
NINE

Your schedule is now complete and I know it has been an extremely time consuming job. Remember, each week you will only be spending 2 hours, but make sure that during these 2 hours you stay focused and work diligently to accomplish your goal. After a few weeks into the schedule you will appreciate your efforts. Trust me on this one! The **RCS** is tried, tested and true!

I hope I haven't misled you when I wrote about the regular cleaning taking approximately 1 hour and 15 minutes and your **RCS** requiring 45 minutes of your time. The figures are correct, but I did not intend that you spend the first hour and 15 minutes doing the once over lightly cleaning then reverting to your schedule and completing the items listed for that week. It is intended that you complete your regular cleaning in each room simultaneously with your week's schedule for that room. If you were to do your regular cleaning and then start with the items on your list, you would be using more time in steps, fetching products etc. and in some instances duplicating procedures.

If you have been cleaning for many a year and have learned through experience the How to's and What for's, you will probably not need to read the rest of this Chapter, but you could humour me.

The following is intended to enlighten those who feel they require further knowledge.

Allow me to take you through the scenario of my cleaning:

Once I complete the mental game, where I say, "It will only take me 2 hours," all I have to do is start and in 2 hours I will be finished, I pull out my schedule and mark the date. (This is covered in Chapter Ten.)

I then go directly to my ensuite bathroom. This is where I always start my cleaning. If the bathroom required only a regular cleaning, then I would clean the sink and counter, then the portion of the mirror over the counter. Next are the shower, the toilet and washing the floor. If I were in Week #3 from **Exhibit # 8-2** (as shown below), I would clean the entire mirror and the lights, then wipe off the artificial flower arrangement before washing the floor and leaving the bathroom.

Week 3 - Baseboards & Windowsills, Bedrooms & Hallways
- Mirrored Closet Doors, Bedrooms & Foyer
- Inside Curio Cabinet
- Bathroom Mirror & Light Fixtures
- Artificial Flower Arrangement, Ensuite Bathroom

Assuming I am in Week #1 of the same Exhibit (as shown following), after doing a regular cleaning of the ensuite bathroom, I would prepare a pail of water with just a drop of cleaning solution (use a cleaner of your choice), but just a drop, as I've previously stated, in order not to leave streaks. I would then start cleaning the bedroom, which would go something like this: wipe all baseboards and junction of the carpet and baseboards, along with areas under the furniture that are too awkward to move, moving small pieces of furniture at the same time; wipe windowsills & ledges; wipe bases of lamps; dust all furniture;

clean mirrored closet doors; vacuum lamp shades, then vacuum the carpet and return moved furniture in the process. The bedroom on this week's schedule would take approximately 10 minutes.

Week 1 - Baseboards & Windowsills, Bedrooms & Hallways
- Mirrored Closet Doors, Bedrooms & Foyer
- Vacuum Chesterfield & Chairs
- Door Frames
- Lamps

If this were Week 2, the bedroom would take 7 minutes or less.

Week 2 - B & W, Living & Dining Rooms & Kitchen
- Mirrored Closet Doors, Foyer & Glass Doors Solarium
- Ceiling Light Fixtures
- Washer Dryer
- Top of Refrigerator

I don't think it is necessary to continue with the remaining weeks; you get the idea.

When I complete each week's schedule, I always have time to walk through my place with a damp cloth in hand and wipe any fingerprints present . You may have fingerprints as a separate item on your schedule, which is fine for a thorough job, but I find that weekly there are only a couple of spots that require attention. *You guessed it...I no longer have children at home.* The other items I do at the same time are individual carpet spots, which have been created in the past week. I seem to have a bad habit of spilling drips of coffee.

Each week I prepare a small dish of carpet shampoo diluted with water and armed with a toothbrush and cloth, I clean these spots. Using this method along with the seven pass vacuuming I can keep the carpet looking like new.

About twice a year I will clean the inside of my windows. When these occasions arise I forego the **RCS**. I do the regular cleaning, then clean my windows and pick up the schedule where I left off the next week. My dust is well under control and my place will sustain a clean look for a missed week of the schedule. *I really did send the dust bunnies packing.*

Another point I would like to make at this time, is never wipe a surface with a dry cloth! You are only moving the dust from one location to another. I find that glass cleaner sprayed directly on a cloth does an excellent job of cleaning items like the furniture, pictures, lamp bases, stove, dishwasher etc. I could go on and on, because I use glass cleaner to wipe everything except those pieces of furniture requiring polish. Glass cleaner is also great for cleaning arborite. It will put an unstreaked shine on smooth arborite and is wonderful for removing stains from a matte finished porous form of arborite. My kitchen counters are this type of finish and appear to stain easily. Kool-aid and tomato-based sauces are the worst offenders. I can spray these stains with glass cleaner and 5 minutes later wipe the stain away. Many of you know this, I'm sure, but I was amazed whenI accidentally spilled glass cleaner on the counter covering a stain that I was unable to remove and when I wiped the area not only was the stain gone, but this area was so much whiter that I had to do the same thing to the rest of the counter. It was great. I love finding new ways of keeping my place clean while saving time.

During the course of writing this book, I asked many people, "How long will it take you to clean your place this weekend?"

The following are some of the responses;

The answer always starts with, "That depends on whether I do a thorough cleaning." Then:

"I've decided that this week my husband is going to do the cleaning. so it won't take me any time at all".

"Well, I don't clean my son's room anymore, so..."

"Well, if I wasn't expecting company this weekend, I wouldn't clean at all."

"Considering that my daughter's room looks like a cyclone hit it...."

"It will depend on how many times I have to stop and bandage the wounds on my ankles from all those dust bunny bites, or should I say dust dragons." This comment came from one of my daughters.

"It kind of depends on how many times I talk myself in and out of the cleaning."

"Considering I will have to stop about twenty times and wipe runny noses and tie shoe laces..."

When all was said and done, the answers fell into the category of 5 to 8 hours, spanning one to two days. A few of the answers were; all weekend.

I hope you adopt my system and never again fall into that never ending category. You will be doing the necessary cleaning every week and only spending 2 hours to achieve a **So....So....Clean!** home.

Chapter
TEN

CLEANING TIPS

Chapter
TEN

Looking at the completed schedule in **Exhibit #8-2**, you will notice that I have left a space at the end of each week. The purpose of this space is to add the date when you complete the individual week's work. Whatever day or evening you decide to do your two-hour cleaning, place the date below the week's work, then the following week you will know the weeks schedule it is time to clean. I have shown my own schedule for an entire year in **Exhibit # 10-1**, at the end of this chapter.

<u>**Cleaning Tips**</u>:(some have been mentioned in previous text).

1. Never dust with a dry cloth. Always dampen or spray the cloth in order to pick up the dust instead of moving it around. Dampen the cloth with water, glass cleaner, furniture polish etc.

2. Never spray glass cleaner directly on a glass encased picture. This liquid could drip under the glass and ruin the 'work of art'. Spray on a cloth or paper towel, and then wipe the glass.

3. Vacuum **high traffic areas** on your carpet with seven passes each cleaning. If a carpet salesman has never told you this, it's probably because he wants you back sooner to buy a new carpet. Any manufacturer will tell you that you will maintain the integrity of your carpet if you go over these areas seven times each cleaning with the vacuum.

4. Do your tidying the day before or earlier. Remember your **RCS** is to clean your home. Tidying is another matter entirely.

5. For the very uninitiated, when you clean bulbs, make sure they are in the off position and cool.

6. If you plan on cleaning your closet, do this before the First Step, as this creates a large amount of fiber dust.

Environmentally Friendly Cleaning Tips

Brass Polish - Worcestershire sauce on a soft cloth.

Silver Polish - One tsp. of baking soda for every quart of water. Bring to a boil, and then add a piece of silver or aluminum. Only badly tarnished items will require even a short boiling.

Rug & Upholstery Cleaner - A good general freshener of cornstarch or cornmeal sprinkled prior to vacuuming will freshen and clean your carpet. For red wine spills pour salt and vacuum when dry. For blood use a thick paste of cornstarch and water pressed lightly into the spot, vacuum when dry.

Oven Cleaner - Moist baking soda in a warm oven will soften stains for easy removal. (Except perhaps Kathy's stains.)

Sinks & Tubs - Baking soda and water will not only prevent scratching, but will leave a nice shine when finished.

Tile Cleaner - Use a mixture of 1/8 cup of baking soda, 1/4 cup of white vinegar and 1 cup warm water.

Lime Deposits - (Kettles, Irons, Coffee Makers etc.) - 1 part vinegar to 2 parts water. Let stand 20 minutes then rinse.

Paint Brushes - The hardest paintbrush can be softened by placing in a can with two tablespoons of vinegar and enough cold water to cover the bristles. Place on the stove, but do not allow to become too hot or boil as this will ruin the bristles. When soft, wash with good soapy water, (The above amount is for a two-inch brush.) or put the paint brush in a baggie and freeze if you are going to reuse it shortly for the same job.

These tips did not originate with me, but have been published over time by our forefathers who did not have the benefits of the cleaning products available on the market today. These have been provided for those who don't wish to use some of the environmentally harmful products on the market and also for those who are thrift conscious.

EXHIBIT # 10-1

RCS FOR A ONE-LEVEL RESIDENCE

Week 1 - Baseboards & Windowsills, Bedrooms & Hallways
  - Mirrored Closet Doors, Bedrooms & Foyer
  - Vacuum Chesterfield & Chairs
  - Door Frames
  - Lamps
  Feb.16; Mar.30; Apr.10; Jun.21; Aug.07; Sept.13; Oct.25; Dec.01; Jan.17

Week 2 - Baseboards & Windowsills, Living & Dining Rooms & Kitchen
  - Mirrored Closet Doors, Foyer & Glass Doors Solarium
  - Ceiling Light Fixtures
  - Washer Dryer
  - Top of Refrigerator
  Feb.23; Apr.06; May 17; Jun.28; Aug.09; Sept.20; Nov.01; Dec.13; Jan.24

Week 3 - Baseboards & Windowsills, Bedrooms & Hallways
  - Mirrored Closet Doors, Bedrooms & Foyer
  - Inside Curio Cabinet
  - Bathroom Mirror & Light Fixtures
  - Artificial Flower Arrangement, Ensuite Bathroom
  Mar.02; Apr.13; May 24; Jul.05; Aug.16; Sept.27; Nov.08; Dec.20; Jan.31

Week 4 - Baseboards & Windowsills, Living & Dining Rooms & Kitchen
  - Mirrored Closet Doors, Foyer & Glass Doors Solarium
  - Shelf Unit Kitchen
  - Stove Exhaust Fan
  - Artificial Flower Arrangements, Ensuite Bathroom
  Mar.09; Apr.20; May 31; Jul.12; Aug.23; Oct.04; Nov.15; Dec.27; Feb.07

Week 5 - Baseboards & Windowsills, Bedrooms & Hallways
  - Mirrored Closet Doors, Bedrooms & Foyer
  - Bookcase
  - Tea Wagon
  - Top of Buffet
  Mar.16; Apr.27; Jun.07; Jul.19; Aug.30; Oct.11; Nov.22; Jan.03; Feb.14

Week 6 - Baseboards & Windowsills, Living & Dining Rooms & Kitchen
  - Mirrored Closet Doors, Foyer & Glass Doors Solarium
  - Spice Rack
  - Fireplace
  - Pictures
  Mar.23; May 03; Jun.14; Jul.26; Sept.06; Oct.18; Nov.29; Jan.10; Feb.21

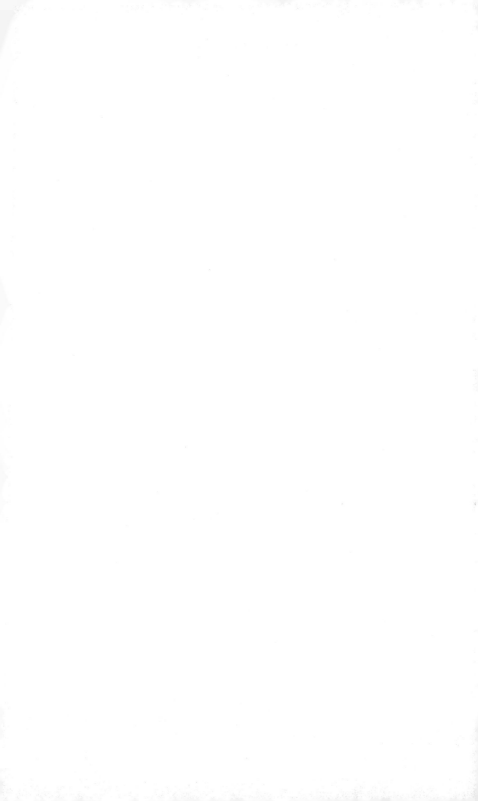

Chapter
ELEVEN

KATHY'S PLACE

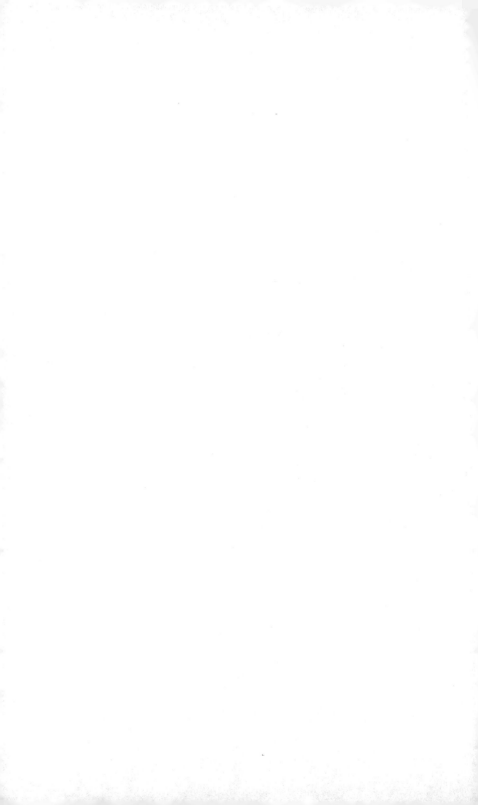

Chapter
ELEVEN

Well, I cleaned Kathy's place! Was it as dirty as she had been saying? Oh, yes! Don't misunderstand me. Kathy's place looked in order; it was tidy and most surfaces were clean, although dull. There was no shine or sparkle. It was dirty!

It took us a few months to set up a Saturday that was convenient for both of us. It's not because we were both so busy we couldn't find any free time. It was probably because Kathy really didn't want me to clean her place. It was the embarrassment, even though she was well aware that I am not judgmental and would not look upon her in any negative way. For me the idea of getting up on a Saturday at 5:30 a.m. to travel two hours only to spend the next 6 hours cleaning..............Well.............!

I cleaned everything. I didn't leave a dust dragon, untouched. I moved every piece of furniture and every book in the place. I've never seen so much dust! I told Kathy, had I known I would have dubbed her Queen of the Dust Dragons, a title formerly held by one of my daughters. In defense of my daughter, she would not qualify for this title anymore; her maturity has taken care of this situation. And, my other daughter now does bedrooms.

It was sure obvious that Kathy hated cleaning.

Kathy had to work on the day I finally cleaned. So I had the place to myself and it went well, a little more than 6 hours. Boy! It looked good! The look on Kathy's face when she came home melted away my exhaustion. As she went from room to room, she beamed like a Cheshire cat.

She just kept saying things like, "Oh!...Oh!." "Oh! My Gosh!" "Oh! My!" "I can't believe it!" "Oh!...Oh!" "This is wonderful!"

For the uninitiated who require more information to complete the First Step, you can find the process I used when cleaning Kathy's place in the addendum located at the end of the book.

Kathy's best words were, "Sit down and don't move. I've brought home two bottles of wine and I'm going to cook you a great dinner." This was music to my ears as Kathy has always been a great cook and an incredible hostess.

Over the course of the evening, we also prepared Kathy's schedule. You will find this schedule as **Exhibit # 11-1** at the end of this chapter. A total of 10 weeks, is certainly a long schedule, but Kathy will still be able to keep a brighter look if she adheres to the schedule. And, let's face it, these items were never cleaned that often prior to the schedule. So, she is ahead of the game.

During the course of preparing the schedule, I mentioned the wall hanging as a 5 minute item.

"Oh, that's something I take down once a year and clean. It does not have to be cleaned on a regular basis", says Kathy.

"Kathy! Kathy! Kathy!" I say. "Have you not heard anything I've been saying? There is no more once a year spring-cleaning. Everything gets cleaned on a regular basis. Nothing is left untouched; your wall hanging attracts dust the same as everything else."

Well! We got the wall hanging on the schedule.

The only time Kathy can do her cleaning is a Sunday morning and the following Sunday I got a call from her.

She couldn't stop talking about the **RCS**. Kathy was tired when she got up that morning and knew that after all my hard work she didn't have a choice; she had to clean.

Kathy is so delighted. The cleaning took her exactly 2 hours and when that was finished, she even cleaned her oven. I just couldn't believe that as well as doing her cleaning on schedule she cleaned her oven. Amazing! Also in a weak moment Kathy said she was almost looking forward to next Sunday when she could do Week #2. I'm not sure, but I think she's getting carried away and I've created a cleaning monster. *Ha! Ha!* This is truly amazing! I really don't think she'll be wishing her week away, but I'm sure that cleaning for her will no longer be drudgery.

Kathy's words for you are, **"Don't even think about it; just do it. You won't believe how easy the cleaning will be."**

Before I close, I have included in **Exhibit # 11-2** a schedule that I once prepared for a woman who spent her days at home, enjoying an early retirement. She wished to do a little cleaning each morning and avoid a 2 hour cleaning once a week. I prepared the schedule and I should let you know that each days work takes 20 minutes to 45 minutes depending on the day. Doing the cleaning daily, in essence, actually takes longer than the 2 hours, as each day you must go through the starting process of getting out the cleaning supplies, vacuum etc., then putting them all away. So, you duplicate this process each day, which during the 2 hour cleaning happens only once. Your schedule, whether you work outside the home or not, may be best suited to a schedule that takes a few minutes each day. The result of this schedule I am told is a home that is constantly clean.

The control over the dust in your home will start to be noticeable in the third week of the rotation. It will take this amount of time to clear the dust that is raised each week while cleaning. Don't be discouraged by dust resettling on your surfaces. Be diligent about your **RCS** and in a few weeks you will see the wonderful results of your labour.

I hope you are successful in accomplishing your cleaning and preparing your schedule. I wish you well.

You too will have a home that is *So....So..... Clean!!*

**Visit my Website at www.sosoclean.com
to print blank exhibit sheets that you
may use to prepare your Final RCS.**

EXHIBIT #11-1

Kathy's RCS

Week 1 - B & W, Bedrooms & Hallways
- Cabinet, Living Room
- Bathroom Wall Tiles
- Lamps
- Light Fixtures Bathroom

Week 2 - B & W, Living/Dining Rooms & Kitchen
- Cabinet, Guest Room
- Bathroom Cupboards, Cabinets & Ledges
- Dining Room Table & Chairs
- Ceiling Fan, Master Bedroom

Week 3 - B & W, Bedrooms & Hallway
- Oven
- Bookcase, Bedroom
- Pantry
- Wall Hanging

Week 4 - B & W, Living/Dining Rooms & Kitchen
- Cabinet, Living Room
- Bookcase, Hallway
- Flower Stand, Kitchen
- Ceiling Fan, Dining Room

Week 5 - B & W, Bedrooms & Hallways
- Cabinet, Master Bedroom
- Chesterfield & Chairs
- Silver Spoons
- Top of Refrigerator

Week 6 - B & W, Living/Dining Rms & Kitchen
- Oven
- Pictures, Bathroom & Hallway
- Ceiling Fixtures Kitchen
- Bookstand on Refrigerator

Week 7 - B& W, Bedrooms & Hallway
- Cabinet, Living Room
- Ceiling Fixtures Hall & Foyer
- Spice Rack
- Milk Can & Lantern

Week 8 - B & W, Living/Dining Rooms & Kitchen
- Cabinet, Guest Room
- Hanging Plant Shelf
- Doors & Doorframes
- Crock Pot & Eucalyptus

Week 9 - B & W, Bedrooms & Hallway
- Oven
- Plates, Kitchen
- Pictures Dining Room
- Stereo

Week 10 - B & W, Living/Dining Rooms & Kitchen
- Refrigerator
- Patio Doors
- Patio
- Pictures, Living Room & Kitchen

Exhibit # 11-2

(This schedule includes the 'regular cleaning' in order to schedule the rooms each day)

Monday
Living Room
Stove

Tuesday
Sunroom
Hardwood Floors

Wednesday
Master Bedroom
Kitchen Clock

Thursday
Guest Room
Microwave

Friday
Kitchen
Bathroom

Monday
Living Room
Refrigerator

Tuesday
Sunroom
Dining Rm. Table/Chairs

Wednesday
Master Bedroom
Kitchen Shelves

Thursday
Guest Room
Baseboards & Windowsills

Friday
Kitchen
Bathroom

Monday
Living Room
Fingerprints

Tuesday
Sunroom
Stereo Cabinet

Wednesday
Master Bedroom
Lamps

Thursday
Guest Room
Microwave

Friday
Kitchen
Bathroom

Monday
Living Room
Front Hall Shelf

Tuesday
Sunroom
Pictures/Mirrors

Wednesday
Master Bedroom
China Cabinet

Thursday
Guest Room
Doorframes

Friday
Kitchen
Bathroom

REMEMBER TO PUT YOUR DATE OF CLEANING BELOW THE DAY!

Addendum
Kathy's First Step

Kathy's place is a two-bedroom apartment with a living room, dining room and a kitchen. I will give you a clue at this point on why it took me 6 hours to clean a two-bedroom apartment. Kathy is an art lover and her living room and dining room walls are covered with artwork from floor to ceiling and wall-to-wall.

I always like to start cleaning at the furthest area from the kitchen and work my way through the place to end up in the kitchen. The last room to be cleaned.

Here we go! (And remember! I am not tidying.)

I fetch the vacuum cleaner and prepare it with the dusting attachment. I prepare a pail of hot water with a disinfectant cleaner and a good size cloth made from an old towel. These are the best cloths for wet cleaning.

I start in the Master Bedroom. The duster attachment is used to remove the dust from a very dusty room.

1.   I vacuum down the drapes, the top ledge of the window frame, the drape rod and the windowsill.

2.   I move all the furniture away from the wall; the bed, two dressers, two night tables, a small bookcase and a chair.

3.   With the furniture moved, I use the duster attachment to go along the ceiling/wall junction to remove any possible cobwebs. I don't stop to look if there are any cobwebs: this would take as much time as doing the job. So, I just do it.

4.   With the duster attachment I vacuum the baseboards around the whole room. I do two things at this point: I remove the duster and use the hose to clean the junction of the floor and carpet (not required for hardwood floors, just use the duster attachment) and I also run the duster over the back of all the furniture as I pass by. And, don't forget the door and doorframe. Because Kathy's baseboards were quite dirty, I go over them with a wet cloth before returning the furniture.

5.   It is time to move the bed back, but before I do I climb up to clean the ceiling light fixture. I remove the shade and wash it with the water I have in the pail. I then wipe the bulb and the attachments with a damp cloth, then return the shade, jump down and move the bed back against the wall.

I will mention to you at this point that if you have a bed without a headboard you should use a wet cloth to wash the wall that is probably stained with hair oil. It may need a spray cleaner on this area to effectively remove all the oil from the wall.

I was once asked by a gentleman, why his furniture was covered with dust an hour after he cleaned. The stock answer for this would be that you have dust in your room that gets disturbed when you move around a room. But, the real answer lies in the question, "Do you clean your drapes and your lamps?"

Its the bulb that is the culprit that attracts the dust, but in doing so not all the dust goes through the opening at the top of the shade, but lands on the much larger and more inviting surface; the lampshade. This is why you clean bulbs!

Let's get back to finishing the room.

6.   The night tables are next. I remove everything visible on each night table including the items on the shelf below. I vacuum the units and run the duster over each item as it's returned to its original place. Don't forget if you have a lamp on your night table make sure you vacuum the unit, shade and bulb.

I will include at this juncture the necessity of cleaning bulbs. When a light is on the heat of the bulb attracts dust. What dust you ask? The dust particles that we carry into our homes on our clothes and hair. When the light is turned off and cools down, then our movement through a room disturbs this dust and it takes flight only to land on you're nice gleaming surfaces.

7.   I now have several units to clean before returning them to their original position: a chair, a bookcase and two dressers. I clean these in the order of the room that returns me to the door. Don't ever waste steps!

a)   I vacuum the chair, front, back and under the cushion, the whole chair. If you have wooden chairs anywhere in your home, wash these down completely with a wet cloth. This wash will apply to any stair railing that you have as well. The pail of water with the disinfectant cleaner comes in handy in every room in the house. I usually change to fresh water for each room. I now return the chair to its original position.

b)   Next, the large dresser. I remove everything as I did with the night tables, this takes less time that trying to move and clean under things. I return the dresser to the wall, it's easier when things aren't sliding around. I then vacuum the entire unit: top, drawer fronts, sides and mirror. I then polish the mirror before vacuum dusting everything before returning them to the dresser.

c)   It's now time for the bookcase. Most people are quite persnickety about the line-up of their books. Some file by author, some file by colour, some file by size and then we have those who file by author while incorporating size and colour into each authors section. God help me! I used to be one of these people. NO MORE! NO MORE! NO MORE! NO MORE! We should write a song: it would probably be a hit. Ha! Ha! So, I am very careful to remove all the books in an order that will allow their safe return. I replace the unit against the wall. I vacuum the whole unit.   I then vacuum the top edge of the books before returning them to the shelves. NOT ONE AT A TIME! I can usually handle about five pocket books in one hand at a time and hard cover about three books.

d)   And, the final item is the tallboy dresser. I follow the same process as the larger dresser less the mirror.

8. I wring out my pail cloth and circle the room removing finger-prints. These are usually found on the doors, doorframes, light switches and cupboard doors.

9.   I vacuum the carpet. Making seven passes over the walking area from the door. I mentioned this earlier in the book that this type of treatment to your carpet will lengthen its lifespan. If you have hardwood floors, you will use your usual method to remove dust.

The total time to clean the Master Bedroom was a ½ hour. One room down and five to go including the bathroom.

I hope you will be able to adapt this process to the other rooms in your home. If I were to detail the cleaning in each of the rooms, much of the process would be duplicated and the information on 6 hours of cleaning would double the size of this book.

I hope you can have fun or at least try to make it fun! Laughing is much better than sweating!